Sugar Detox

Sugar Detox for Beginners:
How and Why to Stay Free of Sugar plus 30 Breakfast, Lunch and Dinner Sugar Free Recipes

Legal & Disclaimer

The information contained in this book and its contents is not designed to replace or take the place of any form of medical or professional advice; and is not meant to replace the need for independent medical, financial, legal or other professional advice or services, as may be required. The content and information in this book has been provided for educational and entertainment purposes only.

The content and information contained in this book has been compiled from sources deemed reliable, and it is accurate to the best of the Author's knowledge, information and belief. However, the Author cannot guarantee its accuracy and validity and cannot be held liable for any errors and/or omissions. Further, changes are periodically made to this book as and when needed. Where appropriate and/or necessary, you must consult a professional (including but not limited to your doctor, attorney, financial advisor or such other professional advisor) before using any of the suggested remedies, techniques, or information in this book.

Upon using the contents and information contained in this book, you agree to hold harmless the Author from and against any damages, costs, and expenses, including any legal fees potentially resulting from the application of any of the information provided by this book. This disclaimer applies to any loss, damages or injury caused by the use and application, whether directly or indirectly, of any advice or information presented, whether for breach of contract, tort, negligence, personal injury, criminal intent, or under any other cause of action.

You agree to accept all risks of using the information presented inside this book.

You agree that by continuing to read this book, where appropriate and/or necessary, you shall consult a professional (including but not limited to your doctor, attorney, or financial advisor or such other advisor as needed) before using any of the suggested remedies, techniques, or information in this book.

Table of Contents

Sugar Detox 1

Sugar Detox for Beginners: 1

Introduction 5

Chapter 1: Reasons to Reduce Our Sugar Intake 6

    How Sugar Affects the Brain and Nervous System 6

    How Sugar Affects the Skin 6

    The Role of Sugar in Tooth Decay 7

    Sugar and the Body in General 8

Chapter 2: Key Benefits of Sugar Detox 10

    Decreasing Your Risk of Sickness and Disease 10

    Empowering You to Take Control of Cravings and Hunger 10

    Boosting Energy 11

    Look Better 11

    Less Cavities 11

    Deter Allergies 11

    Positive Thinking 12

    Getting Rid of Headaches, Aches, and Pains 12

Chapter 3: A Process for Controlling Your Addiction 13

    1.   Eliminate Sugary Beverages 13

    2.   Eliminate Sugary Foods 13

    3.   Search For Hidden Sugars 13

    4.   Keep It Up! 14

    The Most Painless Ways to End Sugar Cravings 14

    What to expect as you detox 16

Chapter 4: Sugar Detox Recipes 18

    Breakfast Recipes 18

    Lunch Recipes 25

    Dinner Recipes 31

Chapter 5: Tips on Staying Sugar-Free 37

Conclusion 40

Introduction

I would like to thank and congratulate you for downloading this book, "Sugar Detox: Ways To Break Sugar Addiction."

Have you ever dreamed of no longer craving for sugar? Living your life healthy and having complete control of your sugar intake? If you are ready to stop your sugar addiction and stop feeling anxious, insecure and depressed, then this book is for you. We will guide you as you start stashing sugar addiction away.

This book contains proven steps and strategies on how to overcome sugar addiction forever. Addiction is something that is easy to acquire yet hard to remove, and most people fail to realize that their love for sugar has become an addiction. To be able to overcome addiction, one must first understand addiction itself and come up with a strategy that will be effective. This book will walk you through a step-by-step strategy, including different causes and ways to break sugar cravings forever, that will significantly improve your health.

The author has gone through everything that you are experiencing. She has struggled in denial and failed many times in trying to remove her addiction to sugar. She is aware that overcoming sugar can be as difficult as overcoming alcohol and smoking. With all that she has experienced, she designed an efficient program for people who lack understanding of sugar addiction and also want to kick the habit. This book will help you figure out if you do have a sugar addiction and help you to overcome the constant sugar craving.

Thank you again for downloading this book! I hope you enjoy it!

Chapter 1: Reasons to Reduce Our Sugar Intake

Aside from unhealthy addiction, there is an extremely long list of reasons to reduce your sugar intake. These reasons range from unhealthy brain function to mood alteration to obesity to avoiding cancer.

Researchers' studies have shown that too much sugar impairs brain function, causes liver damage and obesity, wreaks havoc on our metabolism and could leave us susceptible to diabetes, heart disease, and even cancer.

Unfortunately, with about 80% of our available food containing sugar, it is difficult to avoid consuming unhealthy amounts.

How Sugar Affects the Brain and Nervous System

Some studies have suggested that sugar forms free radicals in the brain's membrane which undermines the nerve cells' ability to communicate effectively. This could affect how well instructions are remembered, ideas are processed, and moods are handled. This can make you seem like a "different person" to those who may know you.

As stated earlier in Sugar Detox, refined sugar is a carbohydrate. In particular, it is a carbohydrate that our bodies are not built to metabolize, especially in large quantities.

Incomplete metabolism of carbohydrates results in forming what is known as toxic metabolites, such as pyruvic acid.

Pyruvic acid collects in red blood cells, the brain, and the nervous system. The toxic metabolites then interfere with the cells' ability to 'breathe,' meaning that the cells are unable to receive enough oxygen to survive and function normally.

Over time, some of these cells completely die off, which ultimately leads to the beginning of degenerative disease. Sugar also promotes depression.

After a six year study of 9,000 test subjects, it was discovered that those who consumed the most sugar were nearly 40% more at risk of depression than those who did not partake in high amounts of the sweet stuff. Bummer.

How Sugar Affects the Skin

Simple carbohydrates such as white bread, refined sugar, and soft drinks, cause insulin levels to spike. This spike in insulin results in a sudden inflammation of the body.

This sudden inflammation produces enzymes that break down elastin and collagen. Collagen and elastin are proteins in the skin which keeps the skin elastic and firm.

When enzymes attack these proteins, the results are sagging skin and wrinkles. Yes, sugar causes you to age more quickly. Not only that, but the sagging and wrinkles are now irreversible.

In addition to increasing the effects of aging, refined sugar also exacerbates pre-existing skin conditions such as acne, psoriasis, and eczema. The more sugar you use, the more likely you are to develop an insulin resistance.

Insulin resistance may manifest as dark patches on the skin in the neck area and body creases such as the armpits. Insulin resistance can also lead to dull looking skin and rapid hair growth – usually in extremely unwanted areas.

Sugar also dehydrates your skin cells, causing redness, puffiness, and circles under the eyes.

The Role of Sugar in Tooth Decay

Poor oral health and sugar consumption go hand in hand. Plaque is constantly forming on your teeth and gums. Plaque contains bacteria which feeds on the sugars you ingest, creating enamel eating acids that start to eat away at your teeth as soon as within 20 seconds of contact.

After the acid eats through even the tiniest microscopic part of the enamel, it starts eating away at the rest of the tooth, causing cavities and tooth rot. Sugar rots your teeth.

The amount of sugar consumed at one time has less negative impact on your tooth enamel than how consistently you consume sugar. If you chug soda, your tooth enamel has more chance of surviving than if you sipped soda over the course of an hour, because the acids have a shorter window to do their damage.

Of course, it wouldn't be such a bad idea to eliminate soft drinks from your diet altogether completely. Why tempt fate? Erosion of tooth enamel can lead to much more serious consequences than just a cavity. Serious erosion can lead to:

- A significant wearing down of your back molars – these are the teeth that primarily allow us to chew our food, whether you're a vegetarian or not. Imagine you're on a fancy dinner date, trying desperately to politely and gracefully chew your food without any back molars. Mashed potatoes, please!

- Tooth loss and extraction of unhealthy teeth – it is an extremely slippery slope. Since teeth are in such proximity to each other and less than sterile living conditions, if one gets "sick," the more likely it is for the teeth on either side to get sick too.

- Extreme changes to your bite – your bite is the way your upper and lower teeth come together. This affects your smile and how effectively you can chew your food, which it also affects your digestion.

- Having to replace damaged dental work – fillings and other dental work have been known to fall out or corrode from the teeth not being cared for properly. Not only can this cause excruciating pain, but it also adds to the inconvenience of taking up time and money.

- Dental implants – if you're lucky enough to be able to afford dental implants, that is. They are highly costly and cause a great deal of pain for a considerable amount of time.

- Gum surgery – surgery. In your mouth. The reason mouth pain tends to be so severe is not only because your teeth are directly connected to nerve endings, but also the mouth is full of all kinds of bacteria that can make the healing process seem like it will never end.

Sugar and the Body in General

The average American spends approximately 130 pounds of added sugar each year. Keep in mind that this statistic includes only added sugar, not sugar that is already naturally occurring, as in fruit or milk.

Sugar adds fatty tissue to your organs, essentially making your organs 'fat'. Added sugars trigger your liver into storing fat in odd places, and the liver does this so very efficiently.

As odd as this may sound, your liver hiding Easter eggs of fat within itself leads to liver disease, a thing rarely seen before 1980 but has, unfortunately, has since become a common occurrence.

A study published in the Journal of the American Medical Association found that those test subjects who consumed the highest amounts of added sugar also showed the biggest spike in bad cholesterol levels and harmful triglyceride blood fats, as well as exhibiting the lowest dip in good cholesterol levels.

One theory is that sugar overload sparks your liver to churn out higher levels of bad cholesterol, while simultaneously inhibiting the liver's ability to clear it out effectively.

Added sugars also cause high amounts of insulin to be released into the arteries. Consistently high insulin levels cause the muscle cells surrounding each blood vessel to grow much more rapidly than normal.

This results in hard arterial walls, which then leads to high blood pressure and makes a heart attack or stroke that much more likely.

High amounts of sugar decrease the hormone leptin's ability to tell your body that it has had enough food, effectively leading to consistent overeating.

Sugar is also proven to starve your body of energy. After a short micro burst of energy, the body goes from sugar rush to sugar crash, because when sugar hits the brain, it triggers the release of serotonin, a sleep regulator.

Chapter 2: Key Benefits of Sugar Detox

Sugar-Free Eating Will Benefit You Mentally and Physically By:

Decreasing Your Risk of Sickness and Disease

Added sugar steals nutrients required for optimal metabolic function. This triggers nutrient deficient disease like osteoporosis, iron deficiencies, and immune issues. Sugar also triggers the growth of hormones with insulin release. Your blood cells are forced to clean up the waste left behind by sugar instead of protecting your body from invading free radicals.

Add this sugar weakens your intestinal tract, so nutrients aren't readily absorbed and dispersed properly. Bloating and gas are notable symptoms.

Empowering You to Take Control of Cravings and Hunger

Nutrient stores are depleted when sugar is on the menu. Some of which are used to help control inflammation. Sugar doesn't contain essential macro nutrients and micronutrients necessary for good health. Good fat, lean protein, and healthy complex carbs are required to satiate your hunger and nip cravings in the bud. Sugar interferes with this and leaves your body and mind unsatisfied and confused.

Sugar is addictive, and you can never get enough. One donut leads to three or four because you are not communicating to your brain that your hunger is satisfied because you are pumping yourself full of foreign substances your brain and body don't know how to interpret or use. It's a cyclical process where your blood sugars get bounced around, and the easy answer is to keep eating more sugar to feel good temporarily. Then when you get dumped to the bottom of the barrel, you crave more sweet stuff to climb out.

Eliminating sugars balances blood sugars, reducing cravings and controlling hunger!

Sharpen Thinking

Scientists have no doubt sugar negatively affects your thought process. Excess refined sugar interferes with memory and fools with concentration. It also triggers negative thinking and unnatural nervousness. When you consume sugar even in small doses, you are altering your brain chemistry. And there's no room for that in healthy living.

Find You, Set Healthy Weight and Stay There

You were born with an internal set weight where your body function optimally. Unfortunately life got in the way, and you likely stressed your body so much your weight reset much higher than is truly healthy for you. By removing the interference of sugar, you will naturally encourage your body to shed fat, assuming you are eating healthy and exercising, so you can find your healthy weight range and stay there.

It's a safe bet that knocking extra sugar out of your diet is going to trigger weight loss fast!

Boosting Energy

WebMD medical expert's state sugar slows you down. When you eat it your energy levels spike. Blood sugars shoot up, and insulin is released. When insulin is released so is tryptophan which converts to serotonin, and sets you up for a nice nap.

By eating a healthy diet loaded with protective antioxidants from fresh fruits and berries, vitamins, minerals, fiber, water, complex carbs, and protein to fuel your mind, you fly through your day instead of riding your tiresome sugar roller coaster of constant ups and downs.

Look Better

Sugar steals nutrients you need to look and feel fantastic. Sugar experts report when sugar attaches to the protein it's called glycation. This takes the blame for wrinkles, saggy skin, and a dull complexion.

Less Cavities
 I'm sure your dentist has told you to point blank that sugar rots teeth. Sugar invites bacteria growth that develops into cavities. Stay away from sugar for better dental hygiene.

Deter Allergies

It's no big secret many allergies are triggered by foreign substances or processed sugary foods. Experts believe people with sensitive systems that subject themselves to extra sugars and processed food additives increase their risk of developing food sensitivities or food allergies.

Positive Thinking

When you are on the sugary moody roller coaster, it's difficult to stay level and focus on the positive. By eliminating sugar, you give your body a chance to find balance in thinking and function. Your constant energized mood will light up your world instead of flood it with dark clouds. The "thehealthyhomeeconomist.com" suggest by 2020 major depression will become a disability with up to 25% of the population suffering from it. Sugar is a direct cause because it destabilizes the brain through glycation. Knock out the sugars, and you have a fighting chance to smile permanently.

Getting Rid of Headaches, Aches, and Pains

Experts agree sugar causes inflammation, and this creates aches, pains, and disease. By reducing or removing sugar from your diet, you'll feel a weight lifted off your shoulders.

Chapter 3: A Process for Controlling Your Addiction

Before you can put an absolute end to your craving for sugar, you have first to learn how to control it. By controlling your sugar addiction with this four-step process, you probably can't consider yourself cured, but you should be able to control your addiction more so than you did before.

Think of this as the third part in ending your sugar addiction: first, you had to know why sugar was bad for you and why it's so addictive. Then, you learned how to come to terms with your situation and admit to yourself that you were indeed a sugar addict. After that, you learned which foods are good and which foods you should avoid. Now, you can learn to control your addiction.

1. Eliminate Sugary Beverages

All of the beverages that were in the no-go zone before apply here. What you'll notice here is that you should focus on eliminating sugary beverages before eliminating the sugary foods. Remember, by eliminating, we are referring to eliminating them during the detoxification process, and then cutting down on them throughout your life. As a general rule of thumb, eliminate all sugary beverages for two weeks before moving on to the next step, which is...

2. Eliminate Sugary Foods

This applies to all of the sugary foods in the no-go zone that we overviewed and discussed in the previous chapter. Start to eliminate the sugary foods from your diet AFTER you have eliminated the sugary beverages. Remember, we want to take this process one step at a time. Resist the cravings you'll feel for more food; a good tip to do this is to treat yourself to other foods you enjoy, but that doesn't have sugar. For example, if you enjoy eating spaghetti (knowing that it's a safe food to eat during the detoxifying process) then eat spaghetti to satisfy your craving for sugar. Soon enough, after a few days, you'll find it easier and easier to resist the sugar.

3. Search For Hidden Sugars

At this point, you've spent two weeks staying away from sugary beverages and another two weeks staying away from sugary foods, and hopefully, you've continued to stay away from them. The next step is to search out all hidden sugar sources. This will require you to do plenty of research and look for foods and beverages that have even a minuscule of an ounce of sugar in them...you may be surprised to learn that many of the foods that we listed as 'safe' actually have a hint of sugar in them. Avoid these foods as well and turn to the true sugarless options for those foods. This process should take another two to three weeks.

4. Keep It Up!

Avoiding all foods and beverages in their entirety that have sugar in them will go a long way to helping you to end your addiction finally, but you can't consider yourself completely cured of the habit yet. You have to keep it up. Those initial couple of weeks we talked about for each of those steps are critically important, but continuing to distance yourself from the sugar is an equally tough challenge. This step may take the same amount of time as the previous three steps on this list, or it may take a little longer. But once you have completed the first three steps and have continued to distance yourself from the sugar, you can move on to the next part of ending your sugar addiction, which we'll examine next.

The Most Painless Ways to End Sugar Cravings

At this point, you know why it's important to end a sugar addiction, you know the foods to keep eating and the foods to avoid, and you've learned a proven step-by-step process for controlling your addiction. Now it's time to end your craving for sugar all together. You may love the taste of a freshly baked pie or a sweet cake, but these are treats that deserve to be saved for when they belong: for an enjoyable treat after a meal or for a celebration of something. They aren't meant to be eaten all the time as normal foods.

While sugar may be an overwhelming temptation for many of us, that doesn't mean it's impossible to put an end to as an addiction. Any one of these methods, or better yet, a combination of several of these, will be the most effective way to finally put an end to your sugar addiction. Controlling it is one thing, as we learned in the previous chapter, but putting the final seal on it is another. Here are the most painless ways you can use to finally put an end to your sugar addiction.

1. Eat Protein Breakfasts

Science is clear in showing that more protein in the morning will inhibit sugar cravings to occur later on. After all, we all remember the popular adage that "breakfast is the most important meal of the day." Focus on eating protein rich foods such as bacon, sausage, eggs, peanut butter, low-fat cheese, and/or Greek yogurt in the morning. These protein-based foods will cause less of the hormone ghrelin to be produced, which drastically stimulates hunger. All in all, making it a habit in your life of eating a protein-rich breakfast will go a mile to ending your sugar addiction once and for all.

2. Don't Skip Meals

By skipping meals, you will become hungrier throughout the day, which in turn means that you'll essentially be making it easier to give in to a sugary snack. Don't fall for this. Eat a minimum of 3 meals a day, breakfast, lunch and dinner, and make sure that those meals are made with healthy foods that will give you plenty of pro-energy carbs and healthy fats. These will keep your insulin and blood sugar levels balanced, inhibiting your craving for sugar.

3. Steer Clear of Secret Sugar Foods

You'll recall that the third step of controlling your sugar addiction in the last chapter was to seek out any 'secret sugars' that you might find in certain foods. Well, if you truly want to end your sugar addiction, you'll have to continue to steer clear of them. If you know of any foods that do have a hint of sugar in them, don't keep telling yourself in the back of your mind that you really don't know about it. Continue to seek out low-sugar foods to keep your sugar intake down.

4. Try Sugar Flavored Foods

Sugar is a very sweet taste, and it can be the desire for that taste that lures you back into eating more sugary foods and putting an end to your sugar detoxification journey. If you find yourself simply unable to resist the taste of sugar, which is the same boat that many sugar and previous sugar addicts are/were in, then you can always turn to the alternative: sugar tasting foods. There are many different kinds of sugary tasting foods out there that actually lack sugar all together. You can put these 'sugar supplements,' if you will call them that, in things such as cinnamon, popcorn, vegetables, and so on. If it's only the flavor of sugar that you appreciate it, then this method will be exceptionally effective.

5. Get Plenty of Sleep

This may sound like an unexceptional way to end your sugar craving, but you'll be surprised at how effective this method is. In order to truly stop your craving for sugar, you'll have to balance two kinds of your hormones: ghrelin, which is what gives you such as strong appetite for surgery, and leptin, the hormone that tells your brain the body is full. Once you can get these two hormones working together, you'll find your cravings for sugar over time go down. Without a shadow of a doubt, the most effective way to get these two hormones working together is to get plenty of sleep, and the current recommended amount of sleeping time for adults is a minimum of eight hours.

6. Get Plenty of Exercise

Like getting plenty of sleep, getting plenty of exercise may also seem like a mostly inefficient way of reducing your cravings for sugar. But if you ever find yourself overwhelmed by your intense desire for sugar, all you need to do is get your body moving. This will stimulate the muscle cells that are sensitive to insulin, which in turn will build up your muscle and produce more levels of glucose. This helps you two ways simultaneously: (a) You'll get your mind off the topic of sugar, and (b) You'll decrease your body's desire for more sugar as well.

7. Relax

Much of the discomfort that results from not getting your daily intake of sugar is just as much emotional as it is physical; you'll recall that we discussed this earlier in the book. You never want to get overly emotional about sugar, because if you do, it can derail the entire sugar detoxification process. Fortunately, you can break this cycle of feeling emotional about not getting the amount of sugar you want. Sit down, take a few deep breaths, and think about what makes you feel like you need to have the sugar. Ask yourself why you are reaching out for the sugar in the first place, and then tell yourself to stop what you are doing, slow down your thoughts, and think about why you need the sugar. Sounds gimmicky? It may at first, but this will actually help you decide if you really want the sugar or if you are just feeding off of your emotions. Sometimes relaxing is all it will take to convince yourself you don't need copious amounts of sugar.

8. Reward Yourself

You can certainly reward yourself throughout the detoxification process, but is rewarding yourself with sugar and sweets the only way to accomplish this? Absolutely not. Think of some ways that you can reward yourself for different tasks. For instance, tell yourself that you'll get some specific things done in two or three hours at work today so you can be more productive. But instead of rewarding yourself with a can of soda or a bag of candy, reward yourself with something different, such as taking a break to think about your dream vacation, or to another kind of food that you enjoy eating that lacks sugar. If you can get on a roll about rewarding yourself when you most need it, you'll gradually lose the thought of sugar in the first place.

9. Take Calcium and Vitamin D Supplements

This one may also sound gimmicky, but it's surprisingly effective as far as sugar detoxifying is concerned. The good news is that if you are currently taking a mineral or multivitamin supplement daily, you're on the right track! Supplements that contain high levels of Vitamin D and calcium will do two beneficial things: lower your weight and decrease your cravings for sugar. Your body's fat holds onto Vitamin D so that your body is unable to use it, but this so-called deficiency actually decreases your levels of leptin. Multivitamins will put more Vitamin D into your body and increase production of leptin. The more leptin in your body, the less hungry that you will feel, and the less craving for sugar your body will naturally have. Granted, turning only to calcium and Vitamin D can't supplement a healthy diet, but they will greatly aid in the sugar detoxification process.

10. Drink Plenty of Water

Surprisingly enough, dehydration is actually one of the major contributors to craving sugar and junk food. Dehydration also has a number of other important side effects, such as lowering energy levels, and causing fatigue, thought inhibition, anxiety, and mood swings. As a general rule of thumb, you should be drinking a minimum of ninety ounces of water per day. However, not all of this water has to come from simply drinking out of a glass. Roughly twenty percent of all the water we consume each day comes from food, such as fruits and vegetables.

What to expect as you detox
The first three days of your detox are the toughest. It does get a little easier after that. You can certainly get through 72 hours, right?

Your tastes will change. After the first week of eating no sugar, you will notice food tastes different. You will be able to taste the sweetness in your bread or your favorite herbal tea. Your taste buds will be more aware of the sweetness in a given food or drink.

The first week of your sugar detox can be physically and mentally uncomfortable. However, it is fairly short-lived, and the majority of the symptoms subside by the end of the first week. Some people report the following side effects:

- Headache
- Lightheadedness
- Drowsiness
- Grumpiness/crankiness
- Emotional
- Pimples
- Rashes
- Flu like symptoms
- Lethargy
- Difficulty sleeping
- Diarrhea
- Constipation
- Skin breakouts
- Gas, bloating
- Body odor
- Bad breath
- More irritable than normal
- Overly sensitive

You are most likely viewing at that list and thinking, never mind. Sugar cannot be all that bad, right? Wrong. Too much sugar can be very bad. Excessive sugar is a serious health issue. All of the above symptoms go away within days or a week. Your body needs time to readjust. Drinking lots of water help in flushing your system and eliminate the rashes and pimples that are part of the detox. The headaches will subside within a few days of eliminating sugar as will the lightheadedness. Again, when that headache hits, try drinking a glass of ice water or closing your eyes for a bit.

The emotional side effects of being a little more cranky than usual will also smooth out. One of the main reasons people abuse sugar is because of the emotional response it triggers. It makes you happy to feed your sugar addiction. It is an escape from what may be troubling you. Depending on the severity of your dependency on sugar as an emotional crutch, you may want to seek out counseling to help you work through the issue that sent you into Sugar's arms.

Chapter 4: Sugar Detox Recipes

When you go shopping for clothes, you take a look at something, and you instantly know you'll look good in it. You have a feeling that whatever you're looking at is the reason you entered the shop in the first place. It doesn't necessarily have to be clothed; it can be anything: mobiles, laptops, hats, purses--anything at all. The point is that sometimes you instantly decide on something because you picture yourself already having it. But how does this work with food? When you see broccoli, you don't picture a healthy you. You virtually taste the veggie and promise to buy it some other time! So say goodbye to that attitude and embrace these awesome sugar-busting recipes to "healthify" every inch of your body!

Breakfast Recipes

1. Protein Muffins (8 large or 12 small)

Prep Time: 10 minutes

Cook Time: 25 minutes

Method:

- In a muffin pan, place 8 cups with paper muffin liners and preheat the oven to 375 degrees.
- In a large mixing bowl, beat together with an egg, two tbs. of canola oil and 1½ cups of unsweetened applesauce with an electric mixer on low speed.
- Now add 1 cup of unbleached white flour, 1 cup of whole-wheat flour, ¾ tsp. of baking powder, two tbs. of unsweetened whey protein powder, ¼ cup of walnuts, ½ tsp. of nutmeg, and ½ tsp. of cinnamon. Beat well on medium speed.
- Add ¾ cup of raisins.
- Spoon the batter into the prepared muffin pan and bake for 25 minutes or until they are well-browned and firm to the touch.

Tip: you can serve these protein muffins warm, topped with organic cream cheese!

2. Apple Cinnamon Oatmeal

Ingredients:

2 apples (peeled and chopped)

8 cups of water

2¾ cups of applesauce (unsweetened)

1½ cups of oats (steel cut)

1/3 cup of sweetener or granulated sugar

¼ cup of butter

¼ cup of milk

4 tablespoons of cinnamon, ground

Preparation:

Right before bedtime, butter the inside of a slow cooker. Combine the apples, water, applesauce, oats, sweetener and cinnamon in the buttered slow cooker. Cook on low heat overnight. Prior to serving unplug the slow cooker and stir in the 1/4 cup of butter and milk.

3. Blueberry Pancakes

Ingredients:

- 1 egg

- 1¼ cups whole wheat flour

- 1 cup of milk

- ¾ cup of blueberries (divided)

- 1 tablespoon of sweetener

- 2 teaspoons of baking powder

- ½ teaspoon of salt

- 10 pats of butter

Preparation:

In a bowl, mix the together the wheat flour, baking powder and salt.

In a separate bowl beat the egg and then add milk and the sweetener. Gradually add the dry ingredients, as you stir until just moist. Fold in the blueberries. Ladle the batter onto a hot greased skillet and cook until both sides are golden brown. Add a pat of butter onto each hot pancake. Divide the remaining 1/4 cup of blueberries and serve with the pancakes.

4. Breakfast Momo

Preparation Time: 20 minutes

Cooking Time: 10 minutes

Ingredients:

- 1 cup almond flour
- 1 tablespoon olive oil
- ½ cup water
- 1 cup shrimp, peeled, deveined
- 2 green chilies, diced
- Salt to taste
- 4 onion, diced
- 1 teaspoon tomato puree

Directions:

1. Cut the shrimps into small pieces.
2. Take a mixing bowl and combine the shrimp with tomato puree.
3. Add in the onion, chilies and season using salt.
4. Mix well and let it stand for 10 minutes.
5. Combine the flour with the water and knead into a dough.
6. Roll it out on a flat surface and cut into rounds using a cookie cutter.
7. Add the shrimp mixture in the centre of each round.
8. Take one edge of the round and fold in to the other side. Seal the edges using a fork.
9. In a pressure cooker pour 1 cup of water.
10. Add a trivet and place a steaming basket on top of the trivet.
11. Add the momo's onto the steaming basket.
12. Cover with lid and cook on high heat for 10 minutes.
13. Serve hot.

5. Homemade Cocoa Nibs Breakfast Cereal

Preparation Time: 20 minutes

Cooking Time: 25 minutes

Servings: ½ cup

Ingredients

- ½ cup chia seeds
- 2 Tablespoon coconut oil, melted
- 4 Tablespoon hemp hearts
- 1 Tablespoon vanilla extract
- 1 Tablespoon Psyllium powder
- 1 Tablespoon Stevia
- 1 cup water
- 2 Tablespoon Raw Cacao Nibs

Directions:

1. Preheat the oven to 300 degrees F.
2. Soak the chia seeds in 1 cup of water in a bowl.
3. Stir and let it stand for 5 minutes.
4. Once the chia seeds have becomes plumped, add in the stevia, vanilla, hemp hearts, coconut oil, and psyllium powder.
5. Mix well and set aside for now.
6. Break the cocoa nibs into small pieces.
7. Add to the bowl and use an electric mixer to blend everything nicely.
8. You should have a dough by now.
9. Use your hands to knead carefully and form into cylinder.
10. Add to a greased baking sheet and bake in the oven for about 15 minutes.
11. Now flip the cylinder dough and bake for another 10 minutes.
12. Let it cool down a bit and cut into small squares.

6. Cinnamon Cream Cheese Egg Crepes

Preparation Time: 5 minutes

Cooking Time: 10 minutes

Servings: 1

Ingredients

- 1 teaspoon ground cinnamon
- 2 egg, beaten
- 1 tablespoon Stevia
- 3 ounces cream cheese, softened
- 1 teaspoon butter

Directions:

- Combine the egg with cream cheese in a mixing bowl and beat until well combined.
- Add in the sugar free syrup, and cinnamon.
- Mix well and set aside for 10 minutes.
- In a pan melt the butter.
- Fry the crepes in batches and serve with syrup on top.

7. Breakfast Protein Pancakes

Preparation Time: 10 minutes

Cooking Time: 10 minutes

Servings: 1-2

Ingredients

- 1 whole egg
- 1 cup almond flour
- 1 packet sugar-free jello
- 1 egg whites

Directions:

1. Beat the egg and the egg white in a bowl.
2. Add in the almond flour and mix well.
3. Add the jello and mix again.
4. In a nonstick pan add one spoonful of the batter.
5. Fry golden brown and do the same with the remaining batter.

8. Blueberry Protein Pancakes

Preparation Time: 10 minutes

Cooking Time: 10 minutes

Servings: 2

Ingredients

- 2 Tablespoon Greek Yogurt
- 1 Scoop Vanilla Protein
- 1/4 Cup Almond Milk
- 1/2 Cup Hemp hearts
- 1/2 Teaspoon Baking Powder
- 1/2 Tablespoon Flaxseeds
- 1/4 Cup Blueberries

Directions:

1. Combine the Hemp hearts with yogurt, vanilla protein, almond milk, baking powder, flaxseeds and mix well.
2. Create a smooth batter and fold in the Hemp hearts and blueberries.
3. Stir gently and heat a sauce pan over medium heat.
4. Create your desired shaped pancakes and fry them golden brown from both sides.
5. Serve with more blueberries on top.

9. Very Smooth and Cool Cauliflower Soup

Prep Time: 5 minutes

Cooking Time: 30 minutes

Serving: 4

Ingredients:

- 1 tablespoon of butter
- 1 crushed clove of garlic
- ¼ teaspoon of ground nutmeg
- ¼ teaspoon of freshly ground black pepper
- 1 and a ½ teaspoons of salt
- 6 cups of water
- 1 chopped cauliflower head
- 1 cubed large sized carrot
- 1/3 cup of chopped green onion
- ¼ cup of chopped fresh parsley

Directions:

1. Take a large sized pot and place it over medium heat
2. Melt the butter
3. Add the garlic and cook for about 30 seconds

4. Stir in the salt, nutmeg and pepper and cook them for another 30 seconds
5. Pour in the water and add the cauliflower
6. Bring the whole mixture to a boil and lower the heat
7. Cover it up and let it simmer for about 20 minutes to ensure that the cauliflower is tender
8. Take a small sized saucepan and place it over medium heat
9. Add the carrots and cook them until soft
10. Add the cauliflower soup to the blender and puree it nicely
11. Stir in the carrots, parsley and green onion and serve hot!

10. The Authentic Depression Era Corn Chowder

Prep Time: 15 minutes

Cooking Time: 45 minutes

Serving: 4

Ingredients:

- 2 cans of chicken broth
- 2 cans of whole kernel corn
- 1 diced large sized white onion
- 3 cups of diced potatoes
- 2 cans of evaporated milk
- 1/3 cup of butter
- Salt as needed
- Pepper as needed

Directions:

1. Take a large sized pot and place it over medium heat
2. Add the corn, potatoes, broth and onion
3. Bring the mixture to a boil
4. Lower the heat and cover it up
5. Let the mixture simmer for about 15-20 minutes until the potatoes are nice and soft
6. Stir in the butter and evaporated milk and wait until the butter has melted
7. Season with some pepper and salt
8. Serve!

Lunch Recipes

1. Tuna Stuffed Tomatoes (2 servings)

Prep Time: 10 minutes

Cook Time: 10 minutes

Method:

- Preheat oven to 350 degrees.
- Drain 5-ounces of low-sodium light tuna and combine with two tbs. Chopped cucumber, two tbs. Chopped red onion, two tbs. Chopped celery, one tbs. olive oil, two tbs. Mayonnaise, one tsp. fresh-squeezed lemon juice, and one tsp. Chopped fresh parsley in medium bowl. Add salt and pepper to taste and mix thoroughly.
- Cut the tomatoes in half horizontally. Scoop out at least 75% of the insides with a paring knife and spoon.
- Fill the cored tomatoes with tuna salad and bake them in the oven for 10 minutes, or until the tomatoes are tender and the tuna is warm.

2. Chicken Broccoli Salad

Prep Time: 10 minutes

Cook Time: 10 minutes

Method:

- Coat a small skillet with two tsp. of olive oil and heat it over medium high heat.
- Chop 4-5 ounces of the skinless chicken breast into bite size pieces and sauté until browned or for about 10 minutes. Stir often.
- In a small bowl, whisk ¼ cup of apple cider vinegar and ¾ cup of mayonnaise together well until thoroughly blended.
- In a large bowl, mix 3 cups chopped broccoli florets, ¼ cup chopped walnuts, 1 cup shredded carrots, ½ Fuji apple cored and chopped, and ¼ cup dried cranberries (no sugar added).
- Pour the mayonnaise mixture over the broccoli mix, add salt and pepper to taste and toss well.
- Add the chicken and toss again.
- Refrigerate for at least 30 minutes and serve cold!

3. Crispy Cast Iron Chicken

Ingredients:

- Chicken Legs or Thighs
- Seasoned salt
- 1 tablespoon coconut oil

Preparation:

Season chicken with salt generously. Set aside for at least 15 minutes. Set oven heat to medium-high.

Over medium-high heat, heat an iron skillet. Add fat. Lightly brown chicken on all sides. Bake in skillet for 35 minutes until cooked through, and skin is crispy. Kill the heat and allow to cool. Serve.

4. The Traditional Grilled Cheese Sandwich

Ingredients:

- 1 tablespoon of soft butter
- 2 slices of bread
- 2 slices of sharp cheddar cheese
- 1 tablespoon of chopped parsley
- 1 teaspoon of chopped basil
- 1 teaspoon of oregano
- 1 teaspoon of fresh rosemary
- 1 teaspoon of chopped fresh dill

Directions:

Spread about ½ a tablespoon of butter on each side of the bread pieces. Place a slice of cheddar on one of the bread pieces (unbuttered side). Sprinkle a bit of parsley, oregano, basil, dill and rosemary on the unbuttered side of the other bread piece. Sandwich the slices of bread together making sure that the buttered sides are facing outward. Take a medium sized skillet and heat it up. Add your sandwich and cook it for 3 minutes on each side until the cheese has completely melted. Serve!

5. Perfect Fat Reduced French Toast

Prep Time: 5 minutes

Cooking Time: 10 minutes

Serving: 6

Ingredients:

- ½ a cup of egg substitute

- 2/3 cup of skimmed milk

- 1 teaspoon of vanilla extract

- ½ a teaspoon of ground cinnamon

- 6 slices of low-calorie white bread

Directions:

Take a bowl and add the milk, egg substitute, cinnamon, and vanilla. Dip the bread slices in the egg mix and coat well. Take a frying pan and spray with some cooking spray. Heat it over medium-high heat. Add the bread slices to the pan and cook them until both sides are golden. Serve!

6.   Mediterranean Tuna Antipasto Beans Salad

Preparation Time: 15 minutes

Cooking Time: 30 minutes

Servings: 8

Ingredients:

- 2 cups beans
- 8 cups mixed salad greens
- 1 large red bell pepper, diced
- 1/4 teaspoon salt
- 1 cup light tuna
- 1/2 cup chopped parsley
- 1 1/2 teaspoons chopped rosemary
- 4 teaspoons capers, rinsed
- 1/2 cup red onion, diced
- 1/2 cup lemon juice
- Freshly ground pepper to taste
- 4 tablespoons olive oil

Directions:

1.   In a pot boil the beans with water for 30 minutes.
2.   Drain well and let it cool down completely.
3.   Add the tuna, caper, onion, half of the lemon juice, bell pepper, rosemary, beans, parsley, half of the oil and pepper into a large mixing bowl.

4. In a small bowl add the remaining oil, lemon juice and season using some salt.
5. Add the lemon oil mixture to the tuna mixture.
6. Refrigerate the salad for 1 hour and serve cold.

7. Grilled Salmon with Tomato and Almond Salad

Preparation time: 10 minutes

Cooking time: 10 minutes

Servings: 2

Ingredients:

- 2 salmon fillets
- 200g cherry tomatoes, quartered
- 1/4 cup flaked almonds, toasted
- 1/2 cup basil leaves
- 1 shallot, diced
- 2 tablespoons olive oil
- 1 tablespoon vinegar
- Salt and pepper to taste

Directions:

1. Season the salmon fillets using salt and pepper.
2. In a pan heat some oil and fry the salmon fillets for 3 minutes on each side.
3. Take off the heat and let it cool down.
4. Cut the salmon fillets into small cubes.
5. Combine the tomatoes, basil, shallots, and almonds, in a mixing bowl.
6. Add the salmon cubes and toss gently.
7. In another bowl combine the salt, pepper, remaining olive oil, and vinegar. Mix well.
8. Add the vinegar mixture to the shallots mixture.
9. Toss gently and serve fresh.

8. Chicken Cashew Nut Salad

Preparation Time: 10 minutes

Cooking Time: 10 minutes

Serves: 2

Ingredients:

- 2 chicken breasts
- 1/4 teaspoon salt
- ½ cup yogurt
- 1 tbsp soy sauce
- Pepper to taste
- 2 tbsp toasted chopped cashews
- 1 tbsp olive oil
- 1 tablespoon fresh lemon juice
- 1/2 teaspoon finely grated lemon zest

Directions:

1. Marinate the chicken using soy sauce, lemon juice, and pepper.
2. Let it stand for 30 minutes.
3. In a grill, grill the chicken for 5 minutes on each side.
4. Cut the chicken into small strips.
5. In a bowl combine the yogurt, salt, lemon zest, pepper, salt, chicken strips and mix well.
6. Finally add the toasted cashews and toss gently.
7. Serve immediately.

9. Coronation Chicken Mango Salad

Preparation Time: 20 minutes

Serves: 4

Ingredients:

- 2 cooked chicken breast
- 4 celery sticks, sliced
- 6 spring onions, chopped

- 1 red pepper, cored, deseeded and diced
- 1 cup apricots, sliced
- 4 tablespoons yoghurt
- 2 tablespoons mango chutney
- 2 tbsp flaked almonds, toasted
- 1 tablespoon curry paste
- Salt and pepper to taste

Directions:

1. Cut the chicken breasts into small cubes and add to a bowl.
2. Add in the celery, spring onion, red pepper, apricots, mango chutney, curry paste and yogurt.
3. Season using salt and pepper and mix well.
4. Add the toasted almonds and serve fresh.

10. Moroccan Chicken

Preparation Time: 20 minutes

Cooking Time: 1 hour

Serving: 6-8

Ingredients

- ¾-1 lb boneless chicken breasts
- 1 tablespoon olive oil
- 1 cup cherry tomatoes
- ¼ teaspoon red pepper flakes
- Salt and pepper, to taste
- 2 red bell peppers, diced
- 1 red onion, diced
- 1 garlic clove, minced
- For the Moroccan spice mix:
- 2 tablespoons olive oil
- 2 teaspoon honey
- 2 teaspoons paprika
- ¼ teaspoon turmeric
- ¼ teaspoon cinnamon

- ½ teaspoon ground coriander
- ¼ teaspoon ground ginger
- Salt to taste
- 1 pinch cayenne pepper
- 1 garlic clove, minced
- 1 teaspoon ground cumin

Directions:

1. In a blender add the Moroccan spice mix.
2. Blend for a minute and transfer to a bowl.
3. Coat the chicken breasts using the Moroccan spice mix.
4. Let it marinate for 30 minutes.
5. In a pressure cooker, add the olive oil, chicken breasts, garlic, onion, bell pepper, and cherry tomatoes.
6. Season using salt and pepper and stir well.
7. Cover with lid and cook on medium pressure for about 30 minutes.
8. Serve hot.

Dinner Recipes

1. Three-Herb Beef Patties

Ingredients:

- 2 pounds of grass-fed ground beef
- 1 tbsp of finely chopped fresh rosemary
- 1 tbsp of finely chopped fresh thyme
- 1 tbsp of finely chopped fresh sage
- 1 tsp of sea salt
- 1 tbsp of solid cooking fat

Preparation:

In a large saucepan, thoroughly mix the ground beef, fresh herbs, and salt. Form into patties.

Heat cooking fat in a skillet over medium heat. Cook the patties for about 5 minutes per side until nicely browned on the outside and cooked throughout. Serve it with any sugar-free sides or bread

2. Lime in the Coconut Chicken

Ingredients:

- 2 lbs of chicken legs
- ½ Cup coconut milk with full fat
- 3 tbsps of lime juice
- 2 tsp of lime juice
- ½ tsp of cumin
- 1 tbsp of garlic powder
- 1 tbsp coconut amino

Coconut oil to coat before baking

Preparation:

Place chicken legs in a zip-lock bag.

With a medium mixing bowl, combine the lime juice, lime zest, coconut milk, cumin, coconut amino, and garlic.

Mix well and pour over the chicken. Place the chicken marinade in the fridge for 3 hours.

Remove the chicken legs from the marinade and place on a lined baking sheet. Rub each leg with melted coconut oil. Bake for 40 minutes until cooked through and browned on top. Serve.

3.   Slow Cooker Beef Stew

Ingredients:

- 3 lbs stewing beef
- 1 tsp onion powder
- 1 tsp garlic powder
- 1 tsp paprika
- 1 lb sweet potato, cubed
- 1 medium onion, chopped
- 4 cups of beef stock
- 5 carrots, chopped
- 1 (16 oz can) tomato sauce, organic

Preparation:

Brown the beef in frying pan with spices. Put beef in the slow cooker along with remaining ingredients. Set on a high temp for 4 hours until well cooked. Serve

4.   Spanish Cauli-Rice with Chorizo

Ingredients:

- ½ pound Chorizo, chopped
- ½ cup Onion, Chopped
- ½ cup of Green Pepper, Chopped
- 4 cups cauliflower rice
- ½ cup Tomato Sauce
- Cumin
- Sea Salt
- Pepper
- Garnishes: Cilantro, Avocado, Lime, and Sour Cream

Preparation:

On a large skillet over medium heat, saute chorizo, onion, and peppers until cooked. Add the cauliflower rice and tomato sauce. Cook until well cooked. Flavor with salt, paper, and cumin.

Enhance with chopped cilantro, avocado, sour cream and a squeeze of fresh lime juice if preferred. Serve

5.   Buffalo Strips

Ingredients:

- 6 chicken breast halves
- 1 cup of chili sauce
- ½ cup hot sauce
- 2 tablespoons of sweetener
- 1 tablespoon butter
- 1 teaspoon garlic (minced)

Preparation:

Combine the chili sauce, hot sauce, sweetener, and minced garlic in a bowl with a whisk.

Add the butter to a skillet and cook the chicken breast halves until no longer pink over medium-high heat. Turn the heat to medium-low and pour the sauce over the chicken strips and cook with an occasional stir for about half an hour. Serve.

Tip: you can sauté the chicken in ½ tsp. of curry powder.

6.   Very Healthy Hot Chicken Legs

Prep Time: 30 minutes

Cooking Time: 30 minutes

Serving: 6

Ingredients:

- 1 cup of garlic chili sauce
- 1 bottle of Louisiana Style hot sauce
- 2 tablespoons of granular sucralose sweetener
- 1 tablespoon of butter
- 12 skinless chicken drumsticks

Directions:

1. Take a medium sized bowl and add the garlic chili sauce, sweetener and hot sauce
2. Take a large sized skillet and place it over medium high heat
3. Add the drumsticks and cook them until they are slightly browned
4. Lower the heat to medium-low and spoon over the prepared sauce, coating the chicken well
5. Let it simmer, making sure to keep stirring it from time to time
6. Keep doing this for about 20 minutes until the chicken is fully cooked and the sauce is nice and thick

7.   The Mighty Lion's Mane Mushrooms!

Prep Time: 5 minutes

Cooking Time: 5 minutes

Serving: 6

Ingredients:

- 1 tablespoon of extra virgin olive oil
- 1-2 cups of sliced lion's mane mushrooms
- A pinch of salt
- A pinch of ground white pepper
- 2 teaspoons of thyme

Directions:

Take a medium sized skillet and place it over medium heat

Add the olive oil and heat it up

Add the lion's mane mushrooms to the skillet and sprinkle over some pepper and salt

Saute for about 2-3 minutes until they turn a golden brown texture

Finish by garnishing with a bit of thyme

Remove them from the heat and serve!

8.   Very Healthy Cauliflower Agrodolce

Prep Time: 5 minutes

Cooking Time: 10 minutes

Serving: 8

Ingredients:

- 2 heads of cauliflower cut into florets
- 4 cups of thinly sliced cippolini onions
- 6 thinly sliced garlic cloves
- 1 cup of sherry wine vinegar
- ½ a cup of parsley
- 6 tablespoons of capers
- Sea salt as needed
- Pepper as needed

Directions:

1.   Carefully blanch the cauliflower for about 5 minutes
2.   Keep it on the side
3.   Take a medium sized saucepan and heat up some oil
4.   Add the onions and garlic and sauté for about 2 minutes
5.   Add the vinegar and lower the heat
6.   Simmer for about 5 minutes
7.   Add the cauliflower and mix everything well, cook for about 10 minutes
8.   Add the pepper and salt to adjust the seasoning
9.   Cook for another 2 minutes
10.   Add the capers for some extra saltiness
11.   Garnish with a bit of parsley
12.   Serve!

9.   Crabby Red Veined Sorrel Salad

Prep Time: 5 minutes

Cooking Time: 5 minutes

Serving: 2

Ingredients:

- 3 pieces of king crab legs
- 2 slices of avocado
- 1 small sized heirloom tomato cut up into 1/8th slices
- 2 ounces of red veined sorrel
- 1 tablespoon of extra virgin olive oil
- 1 juiced lemon wedge
- Sea salt as needed
- White pepper as needed

Directions:

Prepare the crab legs by setting a steamer tray on top of a large pot and pour about 1-2 inch of water in the pot

Boil the water and add the crab to the steamer

Steam the crab for about 5 minutes (making sure to cover the pot)

Remove the legs and carefully crack the shells

Remove the meat and let them cool

Place a slice of avocado on your serving plate, along with the tomatoes and the crab

Dress the crab with olive oil, red veined sorrel and a wedge of lemon

Serve!

10.   Grilled Famous Snapper

Prep Time: 5 minutes

Cooking Time: 10 minutes

Serving: 2

Ingredients:

- 2 snapper fillets
- 1 minced clove of garlic
- A squeeze of fresh lemon

- 1 tablespoon of olive oil
- Salt as needed
- Pepper as needed

Directions:

1. Take a small bowl and add the olive oil and lemon juice along with the minced garlic
2. Mix well to create a marinade
3. Place the snapper in the bowl of marinade and let it rest for about 10 minutes
4. Place the fillets on the grill and cook both sides of them until they are nice and crispy
5. Season a little and serve!

Chapter 5: Tips on Staying Sugar-Free

Once you've completed the detox and decided to move forward with your newfound freedom from sugar, there are a few solid tips on staying sugar-free.

- Mentally prepare yourself for what lays ahead, both the positive and negative. It is so important not to worry; worrying defeats one of the hugest perks of being sugar-free. Instead just realize that you may have ups and downs, and either way, it's going to pay off in a big way.

- Plan out your meals completely. Whether you scribble the meals and their recipes on a scrap piece of paper and stick it to the fridge or prefer to keep a file on your computer, just write them down in one way or another. This will be a big help in keeping you focused and prepared, and leave less room for a lapse.

- Say no. Say it out loud if you have to. This will strengthen your resolution immensely. The more times you say no, and are successful, the easier it will be next time.

- Do not, under any circumstances, ever have sugar in your house. Ever. Period. It would be like a crack head trying to go through recovery in a crack den. Don't do that to yourself.

- Research. There is quite a bit of material out there available to you 24 hours a day on this thing called the internet. Use it.

- Move it! Get out of your way and get all physical and sweaty. Whatever exercise you prefer, make it work for you – and work hard. The natural endorphins your body creates from physical activity make you feel happy and make you want to repeat that happiness. This step is especially critical because you're removing something from your body that it thinks makes it feel good, and it's your job to replace it with something that is. Tough love!

- Take responsibility. It is important to pay attention to what you are eating. Maybe having a cheat day with sugar is not such a bright idea. If you've ever known anyone with an addiction, you know that the concept just doesn't work in the realm of addiction.

- Have fun with your sugar-free self! You are on a great adventure! Move over, giant white whales, swashbuckling pirates, jungle boys, flying nannies, and cartoon princesses – make way for [your name here], who is rediscovering food; and for all intents and purposes, is the brand new owner of a new lease on life. There is a genius in simplicity after all.

- Stock your cupboards and refrigerator to the brim with sugar-free, easy to eat snacks. You will thank yourself. You will miss the convenience of sugar, and since we are used to overindulging, the muscle memory of constantly snacking will be in full force. Having a plethora of sugar-free snacks at your fingertips may be the difference between a slip-up and staying the course.

- Lend a hand. If you feel overwhelmed or underwhelmed or that roller coaster starts to become too much, it is human nature and way too easy to start feeling sorry for ourselves. Instead of wallowing in your sugary misery, lend a hand to your fellow human.

- Try your local food bank or other nonprofits. This will get your selfish 'me me me' brain to focus on 'hi, what can I do for you.' This will lend a lot of perspectives and much-needed objectivity when you may come across people who can't afford to feed their families or get to walk a puppy that is just the cutest fur ball you have ever seen. It works.

- Keep progress reports and know what you are up against. Usually, by the fourth day or so, your sugar withdrawals will be at their strongest. It is difficult not to revert to a junkie mentality, making up ridiculous excuses to those who know your plight, as to why just one won't hurt.

One bite, one scoop, just one. Well, as we all know, there is no such thing as just one. If you feel like you need it that badly, odds are you don't. Your rational brain right now thinks that this sounds dramatic, if not slightly hysterical.

Keep that in mind. Make it a mantra. 'My rational brain knows that I do not need that disgusting sugar, it is hurting me. It is not good for me.' Or whatever you think will work for you. Just prepare yourself mentally for what may and most likely will, come.

It is equally important to equal that out with some resolute positive thinking. 'That will probably be difficult for me but I am strong, and I will feel so proud when I overcome the sugar addiction.' You get the idea...or you will soon (wink, wink). You got this!

- Keep your mind engaged. Play chess or backgammon for the first time this decade. Kick back with a book or crossword. Play minesweeper. If you're a creative type, create!

Just as significant as physical activity is mental activity. The more idle time your brain has, the more it will focus on the fact that it wants sugar. Right now. Now. How about now?

So, maybe refrain from binge watching your new favorite series every day. Maybe save the binge for a reward when you need it. It seems as though binge watching shows or movies is America's new favorite pastime. When most people binge watch, there is usually a plethora of snacks involved. So when you do need to watch for hours at a time, at least make sure you have plenty of those sugar-free snacks close at hand.

Conclusion

Thank you again for downloading this book!

I hope this book was able to help you on your journey into and through the sugar detox, as well as starting your exciting new sugar-free lifestyle.

The next step is to put the recipes and meal plan into practice and make it work for you in the most efficient and personal way possible.

Thank you and the best of luck to you!